Book of Baby Names

A guide to the Origin, Meaning and 1ˢᵗ known use of the most popular baby names

Diego Mendez

Copyright © 2024 Diego Mendez

All rights reserved.

Table of Contents

Boys Names 1
Girls Names 22
Gender-Neutral Names 44
Unusual Names 65
Top 10 Shortlist of Names 83

Boys Names

1. Aaron:
- Origin: Hebrew
- First Use: Ancient times
- Meaning: "High Mountain" or "Exalted"
- Characteristics: Individuals named Aaron are often seen as strong, noble, and principled. They may exhibit leadership qualities and a sense of responsibility.

2. Adam:
- Origin: Hebrew
- First Use: Ancient times
- Meaning: "Man" or "To be red" (referring to the earth)
- Characteristics: Adams are often associated with qualities of groundedness, practicality, and a connection to the natural world.

3. Adrian:
- Origin: Latin
- First Use: Roman times
- Meaning: "Man of Adria" or "From Hadria"
- Characteristics: Individuals with the name Adrian are often perceived as sophisticated, cultured, and possessing a refined taste. They may also be adaptable and diplomatic.

4. Aiden:
- Origin: Irish
- First Use: 20th century
- Meaning: "Little fire" or "Fiery one"
- Characteristics: Aidens are often associated with energy, passion, and a lively spirit. They may also be charismatic and expressive.

5. Alexander:
- Origin: Greek
- First Use: Ancient times
- Meaning: "Defender of the people" or "Protector of mankind"
- Characteristics: Those named Alexander are often seen as strong, charismatic, and natural leaders. They may exhibit qualities of courage and determination.

6. Andrew:
- Origin: Greek
- First Use: Ancient times
- Meaning: "Manly" or "Courageous"
- Characteristics: Andrews are often associated with qualities of strength, reliability, and a strong sense of duty. They may be practical and down-to-earth.

7. Anthony:
- Origin: Latin
- First Use: Ancient times
- Meaning: "Priceless" or "Of inestimable worth"
- Characteristics: Anthonys are often seen as charismatic, confident, and with a natural charm. They may possess a strong sense of individuality.

8. Antonio:
- Origin: Latin
- First Use: Ancient times
- Meaning: "Priceless" or "Invaluable"
- Characteristics: Individuals named Antonio are often associated with elegance, charm, and a love for the arts. They may also have a refined and cultured demeanour.

9. Asher:
- Origin: Hebrew
- First Use: Ancient times
- Meaning: "Happy" or "Blessed"
- Characteristics: Ashers are often associated with positivity, joy, and a cheerful disposition. They may bring a sense of happiness to those around them.

10. Austin:
 - Origin: Latin
 - First Use: Medieval times
 - Meaning: "Venerable" or "Majestic"
 - Characteristics: Austins are often perceived as dignified, respectful, and possessing a sense of honour. They may also have a friendly and approachable nature.

11. Axel:
- Origin: Scandinavian
- First Use: Medieval times
- Meaning: "Divine peace" or "Father of peace"
- Characteristics: Individuals named Axel are often associated with a strong and independent spirit. They may possess a creative and innovative mindset.

12. Brandon:
- Origin: English
- First Use: Medieval times
- Meaning: "Broom hill" or "Gorse-covered hill"
- Characteristics: Brandons are often perceived as charismatic, outgoing, and social. They may have a natural ability to connect with others.

13. Benjamin:
- Origin: Hebrew
- First Use: Ancient times
- Meaning: "Son of the right hand" or "Son of the south"
- Characteristics: Those named Benjamin are often associated with qualities of wisdom, kindness, and a gentle nature. They may also have a strong sense of justice.

14. Bennett:
- Origin: Latin
- First Use: Medieval times
- Meaning: "Blessed" or "Favoured"
- Characteristics: Individuals named Bennett are often perceived as gracious, kind-hearted, and with a generous spirit. They may have a nurturing and supportive nature.

15. Bentley:
- Origin: Old English
- First Use: Medieval times
- Meaning: "Meadow with bent grass" or "Grass clearing"
- Characteristics: Bentleys are often associated with elegance, sophistication, and a refined taste. They may have a love for aesthetics and beauty.

16. Brayden:
- Origin: Irish
- First Use: 21st century
- Meaning: "Descendant of Bradán" (meaning salmon)
- Characteristics: Brayden's are often perceived as energetic, outgoing, and with a lively personality. They may have a playful and adventurous spirit.

17. Caden:
- Origin: American (invented name)
- First Use: 21st century
- Meaning: The meaning is not well-established; it is a modern name with a trendy sound.
- Characteristics: Caden's may be associated with a modern and trendy flair. They may have a contemporary and forward-thinking outlook.

18. Caleb:
- Origin: Hebrew
- First Use: Ancient times
- Meaning: "Faithful" or "Devotion to God"
- Characteristics: Those named Caleb are often associated with loyalty, reliability, and a strong sense of faith. They may exhibit determination and resilience.

19. Cameron:
- Origin: Scottish
- First Use: Medieval times
- Meaning: "Crooked nose" or "Bent nose"
- Characteristics: Camerons are often perceived as confident, charismatic, and with natural leadership qualities. They may have a charming and adaptable nature.

20. Carson:
 - Origin: Scottish
 - First Use: Medieval times
 - Meaning: "Son of the marsh-dwellers" or "Marshland"
 - Characteristics: Those named Carson are often associated with a down-to-earth and practical nature. They may possess a strong work ethic and reliability.

21. Carter:
- Origin: English
- First Use: Medieval times
- Meaning: "Cart driver" or "Transporter of goods"
- Characteristics: Individuals named Carter are often associated with practicality, hard work, and reliability. They may possess a strong sense of responsibility and diligence.

22. Charles:
- Origin: Germanic
- First Use: Medieval times
- Meaning: "Free man" or "Strong"
- Characteristics: Those named Charles are often seen as refined, cultured, and possessing a regal demeanour. They may exhibit qualities of leadership and authority.

23. Chase:
- Origin: English
- First Use: Medieval times
- Meaning: "Hunter" or "To hunt"
- Characteristics: Chases are often associated with energy, ambition, and a competitive spirit. They may possess determination and a drive to achieve their goals.

24. Christopher:
- Origin: Greek
- First Use: Medieval times
- Meaning: "Bearer of Christ" or "Christ-bearer"
- Characteristics: Individuals named Christopher are often perceived as compassionate, kind, and with a strong moral compass. They may possess a deep sense of spirituality.

25. Cole:
- Origin: English
- First Use: Medieval times
- Meaning: "Charcoal" or "Swarthy"
- Characteristics: Coles are often associated with a down-to-earth and practical nature. They may possess a strong work ethic and reliability.

26. Colton:
- Origin: English
- First Use: 19th century
- Meaning: "Coal town" or "Dark town"
- Characteristics: Individuals named Colton are often perceived as resilient, strong, and with a determined spirit. They may possess a sense of adventure and love for exploration.

27. Connor:
- Origin: Irish
- First Use: Medieval times
- Meaning: "Lover of hounds" or "Wise"
- Characteristics: Connors are often associated with intelligence, wisdom, and a charismatic nature. They may exhibit leadership qualities and a love for learning.

28. Cooper:
- Origin: English
- First Use: Medieval times
- Meaning: "Barrel maker" or "Container maker"
- Characteristics: Coopers are often perceived as creative, resourceful, and with a knack for craftsmanship. They may have a practical and hands-on approach to life.

29. Daniel:
- Origin: Hebrew
- First Use: Ancient times
- Meaning: "God is my judge"
- Characteristics: Those named Daniel are often associated with integrity, intelligence, and a sense of justice. They may possess strong moral principles.

30. David:
 - Origin: Hebrew
 - First Use: Ancient times
 - Meaning: "Beloved" or "Friend"
 - Characteristics: Davids are often seen as charismatic, friendly, and with a warm and approachable nature. They may possess natural leadership qualities.

31. Dominic:
- Origin: Latin
- First Use: Medieval times
- Meaning: "Belonging to the Lord" or "Of the Lord"
- Characteristics: Dominics are often associated with a strong sense of leadership, charisma, and a deep sense of spirituality. They may possess a natural ability to inspire others.

32. Dylan:
- Origin: Welsh
- First Use: 20th century
- Meaning: "Son of the sea" or "Born from the ocean"
- Characteristics: Dylans are often perceived as free-spirited, creative, and with a love for exploration. They may possess a poetic and imaginative nature.

33. Easton:
- Origin: English
- First Use: 19th century
- Meaning: "East-facing place" or "East town"
- Characteristics: Individuals named Easton are often associated with a sense of optimism, ambition, and a forward-looking attitude. They may possess a determined and goal-oriented nature.

34. Eli:
- Origin: Hebrew
- First Use: Ancient times
- Meaning: "Ascended" or "My God"
- Characteristics: Elis are often perceived as gentle, kind, and with a nurturing nature. They may possess a sense of compassion and empathy.

35. Elias:
- Origin: Greek
- First Use: Ancient times
- Meaning: "Yahweh is my God"
- Characteristics: Elias is often associated with a strong sense of devotion, intelligence, and a deep connection to spiritual matters. They may possess wisdom and insight.

36. Elijah:
- Origin: Hebrew
- First Use: Ancient times
- Meaning: "Yahweh is my God"
- Characteristics: Elijahs are often seen as charismatic, dynamic, and with a strong sense of purpose. They may possess leadership qualities and a passionate spirit.

37. Elliot:
- Origin: English
- First Use: Medieval times
- Meaning: "Yahweh is my God"
- Characteristics: Elliots are often associated with intelligence, eloquence, and a refined nature. They may possess a creative and analytical mindset.

38. Ethan:
- Origin: Hebrew
- First Use: Medieval times
- Meaning: "Strong" or "Firm"
- Characteristics: Ethans are often perceived as strong-willed, reliable, and with a determined spirit. They may possess a practical and down-to-earth nature.

39. Evan:
- Origin: Welsh
- First Use: Medieval times
- Meaning: "Young warrior" or "The Lord is gracious"
- Characteristics: Evans are often associated with strength, courage, and a sense of loyalty. They may possess a resilient and tenacious nature.

40. Everett:
 - Origin: English
 - First Use: Medieval times
 - Meaning: "Brave boar" or "Strong as a wild boar"
 - Characteristics: Individuals named Everett are often perceived as courageous, resilient, and with a strong sense of determination. They may possess leadership qualities and a bold spirit.

41. Ezra:
- Origin: Hebrew
- First Use: Ancient times
- Meaning: "Help" or "Helper"
- Characteristics: Individuals named Ezra are often associated with wisdom, intelligence, and a deep sense of spirituality. They may possess a calm and thoughtful nature.

42. Finley:
- Origin: Scottish
- First Use: Medieval times
- Meaning: "Fair-haired hero" or "Fair warrior"
- Characteristics: Finley's are often perceived as charming, adventurous, and with a free-spirited nature. They may possess a sense of optimism and a love for exploration.

43. Gabriel:
- Origin: Hebrew
- First Use: Ancient times
- Meaning: "God is my strength" or "God is my hero"
- Characteristics: Gabriels are often associated with a strong sense of purpose, creativity, and a charismatic nature. They may possess leadership qualities and a love for the arts.

44. Grayson:
- Origin: English
- First Use: 20th century
- Meaning: "Son of the steward" or "Gray-haired"
- Characteristics: Grayson's are often perceived as confident, poised, and with a refined taste. They may possess a sense of responsibility and a calm demeanour.

45. Harrison:
- Origin: English
- First Use: Medieval times
- Meaning: "Son of Harry" or "Son of the household ruler"
- Characteristics: Individuals named Harrison are often associated with leadership, strength, and a sense of authority. They may possess a determined and ambitious nature.

46. Henry:
- Origin: Germanic
- First Use: Medieval times
- Meaning: "Ruler of the household" or "Estate ruler"
- Characteristics: Henries are often perceived as responsible, dependable, and with a strong sense of duty. They may possess a practical and down-to-earth nature.

47. Hudson:
- Origin: English
- First Use: Medieval times
- Meaning: "Son of Hudde" or "Son of Hugh"
- Characteristics: Hudson's are often associated with a sense of adventure, independence, and a love for exploration. They may possess a bold and adventurous spirit.

48. Hunter:
- Origin: English
- First Use: Medieval times
- Meaning: "One who hunts"
- Characteristics: Individuals named Hunter are often associated with energy, determination, and a competitive spirit. They may possess a focused and goal-oriented nature.

49. Ian:
- Origin: Scottish
- First Use: Medieval times
- Meaning: "God is gracious"
- Characteristics: Ian's are often perceived as gentle, gracious, and with a calm demeanour. They may possess a nurturing and empathetic nature.

50. Isaac:
 - Origin: Hebrew
 - First Use: Ancient times
 - Meaning: "Laughter" or "He will laugh"
 - Characteristics: Isaacs are often associated with joy, warmth, and a good sense of humour. They may possess a friendly and sociable nature.

51. Isaiah:
- Origin: Hebrew
- First Use: Ancient times
- Meaning: "Yahweh is salvation"
- Characteristics: Individuals named Isaiah are often associated with wisdom, spirituality, and a deep sense of purpose. They may possess a calm and thoughtful nature.

52. Jack:
- Origin: English
- First Use: Medieval times
- Meaning: Diminutive of John, meaning "God is gracious"
- Characteristics: Jacks are often perceived as friendly, down-to-earth, and with a good sense of humour. They may possess a sociable and approachable nature.

53. Jackson:
- Origin: English
- First Use: 19th century
- Meaning: "Son of Jack" or "Son of John"
- Characteristics: Individuals named Jackson are often associated with determination, resilience, and a strong sense of individuality. They may possess leadership qualities and a bold spirit.

54. James:
- Origin: Hebrew
- First Use: Ancient times
- Meaning: "Supplanter" or "One who follows"
- Characteristics: James's are often perceived as reliable, responsible, and possessing a strong sense of duty. They may have a practical and down-to-earth nature.

55. Jason:
- Origin: Greek
- First Use: Ancient times
- Meaning: "Healer" or "To heal"
- Characteristics: Individuals named Jason are often associated with charm, charisma, and a friendly demeanour. They may possess a social and outgoing nature.

56. Jaxon:
- Origin: American (modern invented name)
- First Use: 20th century
- Meaning: Variation of Jackson, meaning "Son of Jack" or "Son of John"
- Characteristics: Jaxon's may be associated with modernity, individuality, and a trend-setting attitude. They may have a contemporary and forward-thinking outlook.

57. John:
- Origin: Hebrew
- First Use: Ancient times
- Meaning: "God is gracious"
- Characteristics: Johns are often perceived as dependable, trustworthy, and with a strong moral compass. They may possess a calm and composed demeanour.

58. Jordan:
- Origin: Hebrew
- First Use: Ancient times
- Meaning: "To descend" or "To flow down"
- Characteristics: Individuals named Jordan are often associated with a sense of fluidity, adaptability, and a calm demeanour. They may possess a harmonious and peaceful nature.

59. Joseph:
- Origin: Hebrew
- First Use: Ancient times
- Meaning: "May he add" or "God increases"
- Characteristics: Josephs are often perceived as nurturing, kind-hearted, and possessing a strong sense of family. They may have a caring and supportive nature.

60. Joshua:
 - Origin: Hebrew
 - First Use: Ancient times
 - Meaning: "Yahweh is salvation"
 - Characteristics: Joshuas are often associated with leadership, courage, and a determined spirit. They may possess a strong sense of initiative and a love for challenges.

61. Josiah:
- Origin: Hebrew
- First Use: Ancient times
- Meaning: "Yahweh supports" or "Yahweh heals"
- Characteristics: Individuals named Josiah are often associated with wisdom, compassion, and a strong sense of justice. They may possess a calm and thoughtful nature.

62. Julian:
- Origin: Latin
- First Use: Ancient times
- Meaning: "Youthful" or "Downy-bearded"
- Characteristics: Julians are often perceived as charming, charismatic, and possessing a refined taste. They may have a creative and artistic nature.

63. Kai:
- Origin: Hawaiian/German
- First Use: 20th century
- Meaning: "Sea" (Hawaiian) or "Warrior" (German)
- Characteristics: Individuals named Kai are often associated with a sense of freedom, adventure, and a love for exploration. They may possess a free-spirited and independent nature.

64. Leo:
- Origin: Latin
- First Use: Ancient times
- Meaning: "Lion"
- Characteristics: Leos are often perceived as confident, courageous, and possessing a regal demeanour. They may have leadership qualities and a bold spirit.

65. Levi:
- Origin: Hebrew
- First Use: Ancient times
- Meaning: "Joined" or "Attached"
- Characteristics: Individuals named Levi are often associated with loyalty, reliability, and a strong sense of community. They may possess a practical and down-to-earth nature.

66. Liam:
- Origin: Irish
- First Use: Medieval times
- Meaning: "Strong-willed warrior" or "Resolute protection"
- Characteristics: Liams are often perceived as determined, strong, and possessing a leadership spirit. They may have a tenacious and ambitious nature.

67. Lincoln:
- Origin: English
- First Use: Medieval times
- Meaning: "Lake colony" or "Settlement by the pool"
- Characteristics: Individuals named Lincoln are often associated with strength, resilience, and a determined spirit. They may possess leadership qualities and a sense of responsibility.

68. Logan:
- Origin: Scottish
- First Use: Medieval times
- Meaning: "Little hollow" or "Small round hill"
- Characteristics: Logans are often perceived as easy going, friendly, and possessing a sociable nature. They may have a good sense of humour.

69. Luca:
- Origin: Italian
- First Use: Medieval times
- Meaning: "From Lucania" (a region in Southern Italy)
- Characteristics: Individuals named Luca are often associated with charm, warmth, and a friendly demeanour. They may have a creative and artistic nature.

70. Lucas:
 - Origin: Latin
 - First Use: Ancient times
 - Meaning: "From Lucania" (a region in Southern Italy)
 - Characteristics: Lucas is often perceived as charismatic, kind-hearted, and possessing a strong sense of empathy. They may have a calm and composed nature.

71. Luke:
- Origin: Greek
- First Use: Ancient times
- Meaning: "Light-giving" or "Bringer of light"
- Characteristics: Individuals named Luke are often associated with intelligence, kindness, and a gentle demeanour. They may possess a calm and thoughtful nature.

72. Mason:
- Origin: English
- First Use: Medieval times
- Meaning: "Worker in stone" or "Stone mason"
- Characteristics: Masons are often perceived as practical, dependable, and possessing a strong work ethic. They may have a determined and focused nature.

73. Mateo:
- Origin: Spanish
- First Use: Medieval times
- Meaning: "Gift of God"
- Characteristics: Mateos are often associated with charm, warmth, and a friendly demeanour. They may have a strong sense of empathy and compassion.

74. Matthew:
- Origin: Hebrew
- First Use: Ancient times
- Meaning: "Gift of God"
- Characteristics: Matthews are often perceived as reliable, responsible, and possessing a strong sense of duty. They may have a practical and down-to-earth nature.

75. Maverick:
- Origin: American
- First Use: 19th century
- Meaning: "Independent" or "Unorthodox"
- Characteristics: Mavericks are often associated with independence, creativity, and a free-spirited nature. They may possess a bold and adventurous spirit.

76. Max:
- Origin: Latin
- First Use: Ancient times
- Meaning: "Greatest" or "The greatest"
- Characteristics: Maxes are often perceived as confident, ambitious, and possessing a strong sense of leadership. They may have a competitive and determined nature.

77. Michael:
- Origin: Hebrew
- First Use: Ancient times
- Meaning: "Who is like God?"
- Characteristics: Michaels are often associated with strength, courage, and a sense of protection. They may have a caring and nurturing nature.

78. Miles:
- Origin: Latin
- First Use: Medieval times
- Meaning: "Soldier" or "Merciful"
- Characteristics: Miles are often perceived as disciplined, determined, and possessing a strong sense of duty. They may have a focused and goal-oriented nature.

79. Nathan:
- Origin: Hebrew
- First Use: Ancient times
- Meaning: "He has given" or "Gift from God"
- Characteristics: Nathans are often associated with wisdom, intelligence, and a deep sense of spirituality. They may have a calm and thoughtful nature.

80. Nathaniel:
 - Origin: Hebrew
 - First Use: Ancient times
 - Meaning: "Gift of God"
 - Characteristics: Nathaniels are often perceived as kind-hearted, compassionate, and possessing a strong sense of empathy. They may have a gentle and caring nature.

81. Nicholas:
- Origin: Greek
- First Use: Ancient times
- Meaning: "Victory of the people"
- Characteristics: Individuals named Nicholas are often associated with generosity, kindness, and a warm-hearted nature. They may possess a charismatic and friendly demeanour.

82. Noah:
- Origin: Hebrew
- First Use: Ancient times
- Meaning: "Rest" or "Comfort"
- Characteristics: Noah's are often perceived as gentle, calm, and possessing a nurturing nature. They may have a strong sense of empathy and compassion.

83. Nolan:
- Origin: Irish
- First Use: 20th century
- Meaning: "Champion" or "Noble one"
- Characteristics: Nolans are often associated with determination, resilience, and a strong sense of individuality. They may possess leadership qualities and a bold spirit.

84. Oliver:
- Origin: Latin
- First Use: Medieval times
- Meaning: "Olive tree" or "Peaceful"
- Characteristics: Olivers are often perceived as refined, charming, and possessing a love for aesthetics. They may have a creative and artistic nature.

85. Owen:
- Origin: Welsh
- First Use: Medieval times
- Meaning: "Young warrior" or "Well-born"
- Characteristics: Owens are often associated with strength, courage, and a sense of loyalty. They may possess a resilient and tenacious nature.

86. Pedro:
- Origin: Spanish, Portuguese
- First Use: Medieval times
- Meaning: "Rock" or "stone"
- Characteristics: Pedro is a classic name associated with strength, solidity, and dependability. Individuals named Pedro are often seen as resilient and steadfast. The name has biblical and cultural significance, especially in Spanish and Portuguese-speaking regions.

87. Robert:
- Origin: Germanic
- First Use: Medieval times
- Meaning: "Bright fame" or "Famous one"
- Characteristics: Roberts are often associated with reliability, responsibility, and a strong work ethic. They may possess a practical and down-to-earth nature.

88. Roman:
- Origin: Latin
- First Use: Ancient times
- Meaning: "Citizen of Rome"
- Characteristics: Romans are often perceived as strong-willed, confident, and possessing a bold spirit. They may have a natural affinity for leadership.

89. Ryan:
- Origin: Irish
- First Use: Medieval times
- Meaning: "Little king" or "Kingly"
- Characteristics: Ryans are often associated with charisma, friendliness, and a sociable nature. They may possess a warm and approachable demeanour.

90. Ryder:
 - Origin: English
 - First Use: 20th century
 - Meaning: "Horseman" or "Knight"
 - Characteristics: Ryders are often perceived as adventurous, independent, and possessing a free-spirited nature. They may have a love for exploration and a bold attitude.

91. Samuel:
- Origin: Hebrew
- First Use: Ancient times
- Meaning: "Heard by God" or "Name of God"
- Characteristics: Samuels are often associated with wisdom, humility, and a gentle demeanour. They may possess a calm and thoughtful nature.

92. Saul:
- Origin: Hebrew
- First Use: Ancient times
- Meaning: "Asked for" or "prayed for"
- Characteristics: Saul is a name with biblical origins, associated with someone who is requested or desired. Individuals with this name may be seen as determined, purposeful, and deeply connected to their roots.

93. Sebastian:
- Origin: Latin
- First Use: Ancient times
- Meaning: "Venerable" or "Revered"
- Characteristics: Sebastians are often associated with charm, sophistication, and a refined taste. They may have a creative and artistic nature.

94. Theodore:
- Origin: Greek
- First Use: Ancient times
- Meaning: "God's gift" or "Gift of God"
- Characteristics: Theodores are often perceived as compassionate, kind-hearted, and possessing a strong sense of empathy. They may have a nurturing and caring nature.

95. Thomas:
- Origin: Aramaic
- First Use: Ancient times
- Meaning: "Twin"
- Characteristics: Thomases are often associated with intelligence, curiosity, and a love for learning. They may possess a thoughtful and analytical nature.

96. Wesley:
- Origin: English
- First Use: Medieval times
- Meaning: "Western meadow" or "Western clearing"
- Characteristics: Wesley's are often perceived as friendly, outgoing, and possessing a sociable nature. They may have a love for community and social interactions.

97. William:
- Origin: Germanic
- First Use: Medieval times
- Meaning: "Resolute protector" or "Strong-willed warrior"
- Characteristics: Williams are often associated with strength, leadership, and a sense of responsibility. They may possess a determined and ambitious nature.

98. Wyatt:
- Origin: English
- First Use: Medieval times
- Meaning: "Brave in war" or "Hardy"
- Characteristics: Wyatts are often perceived as courageous, resilient, and possessing a determined spirit. They may have a strong sense of individuality.

99. Xavier:
- Origin: Basque
- First Use: Medieval times
- Meaning: "New house" or "Bright"
- Characteristics: Xaviers are often associated with charisma, intelligence, and a strong sense of individuality. They may possess a bold and adventurous spirit.

100.   Zachary:
 - Origin: Hebrew
 - First Use: Medieval times
 - Meaning: "Yahweh remembers"
 - Characteristics: Zachary's are often perceived as friendly, sociable, and possessing a warm-hearted nature. They may have a good sense of humour and a love for social interactions.

101.   Zayden:
 - Origin: Modern invented name
 - First Use: 21st century
 - Meaning: Combination of modern sounds
 - Characteristics: Zayden's may be associated with modernity, uniqueness, and a trend-setting attitude. They may have a contemporary and forward-thinking outlook.

Girls Names

1. Aaliyah:
- Origin: Arabic
- First Use: Late 20th century
- Meaning: "Exalted" or "High"
- Characteristics: Aaliyahs are often associated with grace, elegance, and a strong sense of individuality. They may possess a calm and composed nature.

2. Abigail:
- Origin: Hebrew
- First Use: Medieval times
- Meaning: "Father's joy" or "Joy of the father"
- Characteristics: Abigails are often perceived as kind-hearted, nurturing, and possessing a warm demeanour. They may have a strong sense of empathy.

3. Adeline:
- Origin: Germanic
- First Use: Medieval times
- Meaning: "Noble" or "Noble natured"
- Characteristics: Adelines are often perceived as refined, sophisticated, and possessing a love for aesthetics. They may have a creative and artistic nature.

4. Alice:
- Origin: Germanic
- First Use: Medieval times
- Meaning: "Noble" or "Of noble birth"
- Characteristics: Alices are often perceived as intelligent, curious, and possessing a love for learning. They may have a thoughtful and analytical nature.

5. Alison:
- Origin: Old French
- First Use: Medieval times
- Meaning: "Noble" or "Of noble birth"
- Characteristics: Alisons are often associated with kindness, compassion, and a warm-hearted nature. They may possess a strong sense of community.

6. Amelia:
- Origin: Germanic
- First Use: Medieval times
- Meaning: "Work" or "Industrious"
- Characteristics: Amelias are often perceived as diligent, responsible, and possessing a strong work ethic. They may have a determined and ambitious nature.

7. Angelina:
- Origin: Greek
- First Use: Medieval times
- Meaning: "Messenger of God" or "Angelic"
- Characteristics: Angelinas are often associated with grace, beauty, and a gentle demeanour. They may possess a nurturing and caring nature.

8. Aria:
 - Origin: Italian
 - First Use: 20th century
 - Meaning: "Air" or "Melody"

- Characteristics: Arias are often perceived as creative, expressive, and possessing a love for the arts. They may have a free-spirited and independent nature.

9. Ariana:
- Origin: Italian
- First Use: Medieval times
- Meaning: "Most holy" or "Very holy"
- Characteristics: Arianas are often associated with elegance, sophistication, and a love for beauty. They may possess a creative and artistic nature.

10. Ariel:
- Origin: Hebrew
- First Use: Medieval times
- Meaning: "Lion of God" or "Lioness of God"
- Characteristics: Ariels are often perceived as independent, strong-willed, and possessing a free-spirited nature. They may have a love for adventure.

11. Athena:
- Origin: Greek
- First Use: Ancient times
- Meaning: "Goddess of wisdom" or "Wise"
- Characteristics: Athenas are often associated with intelligence, wisdom, and a strong sense of justice. They may possess leadership qualities.

12. Aubrey:
- Origin: Germanic
- First Use: Medieval times
- Meaning: "Noble ruler" or "Elf ruler"
- Characteristics: Aubrey's are often perceived as charming, sociable, and possessing a friendly demeanour. They may have a love for social interactions.

13. Audrey:
- Origin: Old English
- First Use: Medieval times
- Meaning: "Noble strength" or "Noble one"
- Characteristics: Audreys are often associated with grace, strength, and a refined taste. They may possess a calm and composed nature.

14. Aurora:
- Origin: Latin
- First Use: Ancient times
- Meaning: "Dawn" or "Goddess of the dawn"
- Characteristics: Auroras are often perceived as vibrant, optimistic, and possessing a joyful nature. They may have a love for beauty and the arts.

15. Autumn:
- Origin: Latin
- First Use: Medieval times
- Meaning: "Fall season" or "Harvest"
- Characteristics: Autumns are often associated with warmth, creativity, and a nurturing nature. They may possess a love for nature and the changing seasons.

16. Ava:
- Origin: Germanic
- First Use: Medieval times
- Meaning: "Life" or "Living one"
- Characteristics: Avas are often perceived as graceful, elegant, and possessing a timeless beauty. They may have a gentle and compassionate nature.

17. Avery:
- Origin: Old English
- First Use: Medieval times
- Meaning: "Ruler of the elves" or "Elf counsellor"

- Characteristics: Averys are often associated with creativity, individuality, and a love for self-expression. They may possess a bold and adventurous spirit.

18. Bella:
 - Origin: Italian
 - First Use: Medieval times
 - Meaning: "Beautiful" or "Lovely"
 - Characteristics: Bellas are often perceived as charming, graceful, and possessing a captivating presence. They may have a love for aesthetics and a gentle demeanour.

19. Brielle:
- Origin: French
- First Use: 20th century
- Meaning: "God is my strength" or "Strong"
- Characteristics: Brielle's are often associated with strength, resilience, and a determined spirit. They may possess a warm and caring nature.

20. Brooklyn:
- Origin: Dutch
- First Use: 19th century
- Meaning: "Water" or "Stream"
- Characteristics: Brooklyn's are often perceived as independent, adventurous, and possessing a free-spirited nature. They may have a love for exploration.

21. Camila:
- Origin: Latin
- First Use: Ancient times
- Meaning: "Free-born" or "Noble"
- Characteristics: Camilas are often associated with elegance, grace, and a refined taste. They may possess a love for aesthetics and beauty.

22. Caroline:
- Origin: French
- First Use: Medieval times

- Meaning: "Free man" or "Strong"
- Characteristics: Carolines are often perceived as charming, sociable, and possessing a warm demeanour. They may have a love for social interactions.

23. Chloe:
- Origin: Greek
- First Use: Ancient times
- Meaning: "Young green shoot" or "Blooming"
- Characteristics: Chloes are often associated with youthfulness, vitality, and a vibrant spirit. They may possess a cheerful and optimistic nature.

24. Claire:
- Origin: French
- First Use: Medieval times
- Meaning: "Clear" or "Bright"
- Characteristics: Claires are often perceived as clear-thinking, intelligent, and possessing a calm demeanour. They may have a love for clarity and simplicity.

25. Clara:
- Origin: Latin
- First Use: Medieval times
- Meaning: "Clear" or "Bright"
- Characteristics: Claras are often associated with clarity, grace, and a refined taste. They may possess a creative and artistic nature.

26. Eleanor:
- Origin: Greek
- First Use: Medieval times
- Meaning: "Bright, shining one" or "Sun ray"
- Characteristics: Eleanors are often perceived as wise, charismatic, and possessing a strong sense of leadership. They may have a nurturing and caring nature.

27. Ella:
- Origin: Old German

- First Use: Medieval times
- Meaning: "Fairy maiden" or "Beautiful fairy"
- Characteristics: Ellas are often associated with beauty, grace, and a gentle demeanour. They may possess a kind and compassionate nature.

28. Ellie:
 - Origin: English
 - First Use: Medieval times
 - Meaning: "Short form of Eleanor" or "Shining light"
 - Characteristics: Ellies are often perceived as joyful, friendly, and possessing a warm-hearted nature. They may have a playful and optimistic outlook.

29. Eloise:
- Origin: Old French
- First Use: Medieval times
- Meaning: "Healthy" or "Wide"
- Characteristics: Eloises are often associated with elegance, charm, and a refined taste. They may possess a sophisticated and creative nature.

30. Elsie:
- Origin: Scottish
- First Use: Medieval times
- Meaning: "Noble" or "God is my oath"
- Characteristics: Elsies are often perceived as sweet, charming, and possessing a gentle demeanour. They may have a love for simplicity.

31. Emery:
- Origin: Germanic
- First Use: Medieval times
- Meaning: "Brave" or "Industrious"
- Characteristics: Emerys are often associated with strength, resilience, and a determined spirit. They may possess a warm and caring nature.

32. Emily:
- Origin: Latin
- First Use: Medieval times

- Meaning: "Rival" or "Industrious"
- Characteristics: Emilys are often perceived as intelligent, diligent, and possessing a strong work ethic. They may have a warm and friendly nature.

33. Emma:
- Origin: Germanic
- First Use: Medieval times
- Meaning: "Whole" or "Universal"
- Characteristics: Emma's are often associated with warmth, kindness, and a nurturing nature. They may possess a timeless and classic charm.

34. Eva:
- Origin: Hebrew
- First Use: Medieval times
- Meaning: "Life" or "Living one"
- Characteristics: Eva's are often perceived as graceful, elegant, and possessing a timeless beauty. They may have a gentle and compassionate nature.

35. Evelyn:
- Origin: Old English
- First Use: Medieval times
- Meaning: "Desired" or "Wished for"
- Characteristics: Evelyns are often associated with elegance, charm, and a love for aesthetics. They may possess a sophisticated and creative nature.

36. Everlee (and Everly):
- Origin: English
- First Use: 21st century
- Meaning: "Forever meadow" or "Always field"
- Characteristics: Everlee's are often perceived as free-spirited, nature-loving, and possessing a gentle demeanour. They may have a love for tranquillity.

37. Gabriella:
- Origin: Italian
- First Use: Medieval times
- Meaning: "God is my strength" or "Strong"
- Characteristics: Gabrielles are often associated with strength, resilience, and a determined spirit. They may possess a warm and caring nature.

38. Grace:
- Origin: Latin
- First Use: Medieval times
- Meaning: "Grace" or "Favor"
- Characteristics: Graces are often perceived as elegant, charming, and possessing a gentle demeanour. They may have a timeless and classic charm.

39. Hailey:
- Origin: English
- First Use: 20th century
- Meaning: "Hay meadow" or "Hay clearing"
- Characteristics: Haileys are often perceived as cheerful, friendly, and possessing a warm-hearted nature. They may have a playful and optimistic outlook.

40. Hannah:
- Origin: Hebrew
- First Use: Medieval times
- Meaning: "Grace" or "Favor"
- Characteristics: Hannahs are often associated with kindness, compassion, and a warm demeanour. They may possess a strong sense of empathy.

41. Hazel:
- Origin: English
- First Use: Medieval times
- Meaning: "Hazel tree" or "Light brown"

- Characteristics: Hazels are often associated with warmth, creativity, and a nurturing nature. They may possess a love for nature and the changing seasons.

42. Hope:
- Origin: English
- First Use: 17th century
- Meaning: "Hope" or "Trust"
- Characteristics: Hopes are often perceived as optimistic, positive, and possessing a resilient spirit. They may have a strong sense of determination.

43. Isabel:
- Origin: Spanish
- First Use: Medieval times
- Meaning: "God is my oath" or "Consecrated to God"
- Characteristics: Isabels are often associated with elegance, charm, and a refined taste. They may possess a sophisticated and creative nature.

44. Isabella:
 - Origin: Italian
 - First Use: Medieval times
 - Meaning: "God is my oath" or "Consecrated to God"
 - Characteristics: Isabellas are often perceived as graceful, elegant, and possessing a timeless beauty. They may have a gentle and compassionate nature.

45. Isla:
- Origin: Scottish
- First Use: Medieval times
- Meaning: "Island" or "Dweller on an island"
- Characteristics: Islas are often associated with tranquillity, a love for nature, and a calm demeanour. They may possess a gentle and nurturing nature.

46. Ivy:
- Origin: Old English

- First Use: Medieval times
- Meaning: "Climbing vine" or "Faithfulness"
- Characteristics: Ivys are often perceived as resilient, adaptable, and possessing a strong sense of loyalty. They may have a love for growth and transformation.

47. Jade:
- Origin: Spanish
- First Use: 19th century
- Meaning: "Green gemstone" or "Precious stone"
- Characteristics: Jades are often associated with elegance, beauty, and a refined taste. They may possess a calm and composed nature.

48. Jasmine:
- Origin: Persian
- First Use: Medieval times
- Meaning: "Gift from God" or "Jasminum flower"
- Characteristics: Jasmines are often perceived as graceful, charming, and possessing a gentle demeanour. They may have a love for beauty and grace.

49. Josephine:
- Origin: French
- First Use: 19th century
- Meaning: "God will add" or "God increases"
- Characteristics: Josephines are often associated with grace, elegance, and a refined taste. They may possess a sophisticated and creative nature.

50. Katherine:
- Origin: Greek
- First Use: Medieval times
- Meaning: "Pure" or "Clear"
- Characteristics: Katherines are often perceived as intelligent, confident, and possessing a strong sense of leadership. They may have a nurturing and caring nature.

51. Kaylee:
- Origin: Irish
- First Use: 20th century
- Meaning: "Pure" or "Slim and fair"
- Characteristics: Kaylee's are often associated with a playful and cheerful nature. They may possess a love for laughter and enjoyment.

52. Kennedy:
- Origin: Irish
- First Use: 20th century
- Meaning: "Helmeted chief" or "Misshapen head"
- Characteristics: Kennedys are often perceived as confident, ambitious, and possessing a strong sense of determination. They may have a leadership-oriented nature.

53. Layla:
- Origin: Arabic
- First Use: Medieval times
- Meaning: "Night" or "Dark beauty"
- Characteristics: Laylas are often associated with mystery, beauty, and a gentle demeanour. They may possess a calm and composed nature.

54. Leah:
 - Origin: Hebrew
 - First Use: Medieval times
 - Meaning: "Weary" or "Gazelle"
 - Characteristics: Leahs are often perceived as kind-hearted, nurturing, and possessing a warm demeanour. They may have a strong sense of empathy.

55. Leilani:
- Origin: Hawaiian
- First Use: 20th century
- Meaning: "Heavenly flowers" or "Royal child"
- Characteristics: Leilanis are often associated with grace, beauty, and a love for nature. They may possess a gentle and nurturing nature.

56. Lila:
- Origin: Arabic
- First Use: Medieval times
- Meaning: "Night" or "Dark beauty"
- Characteristics: Lilas are often perceived as mysterious, elegant, and possessing a gentle demeanour. They may have a calm and composed nature.

57. Lillian:
- Origin: Latin
- First Use: Medieval times
- Meaning: "Lily" or "Pure"
- Characteristics: Lillians are often associated with purity, grace, and a timeless beauty. They may possess a sophisticated and refined taste.

58. Lily:
- Origin: English
- First Use: Medieval times
- Meaning: "Lily flower" or "Pure"
- Characteristics: Lilys are often perceived as pure, graceful, and possessing a timeless beauty. They may have a gentle and nurturing nature.

59. Lucy:
- Origin: Latin
- First Use: Medieval times
- Meaning: "Light" or "Bringer of light"
- Characteristics: Lucys are often associated with brightness, intelligence, and a warm demeanour. They may possess a friendly and sociable nature.

60. Luna:
- Origin: Latin
- First Use: Ancient times
- Meaning: "Moon" or "Goddess of the moon"

- Characteristics: Lunas are often perceived as mystical, gentle, and possessing a calm demeanour. They may have a love for introspection and spirituality.

61. Madeline:
- Origin: English
- First Use: Medieval times
- Meaning: "High tower" or "Woman of Magdala"
- Characteristics: Madeline's are often associated with elegance, grace, and a refined taste. They may possess a sophisticated and creative nature.

62. Madelyn:
- Origin: English
- First Use: 19th century
- Meaning: "High tower" or "Woman of Magdala"
- Characteristics: Madelyn's are often perceived as confident, intelligent, and possessing a strong sense of leadership. They may have a nurturing and caring nature.

63. Madison:
- Origin: English
- First Use: 19th century
- Meaning: "Son of Maud" or "Gift of God"
- Characteristics: Madisons are often associated with confidence, ambition, and a strong sense of determination. They may have a leadership-oriented nature.

64. Makenzie:
- Origin: Scottish
- First Use: 20th century
- Meaning: "Son of the wise leader" or "Fair one"
- Characteristics: Makenzie's are often perceived as wise, fair-minded, and possessing a warm demeanour. They may have a love for knowledge and fairness.

65. Megan:
- Origin: Welsh
- First Use: 20th century
- Meaning: "Pearl" or "Little pearl"
- Characteristics: Megans are often associated with purity, elegance, and a gentle demeanour. They may possess a warm and caring nature.

66. Mia:
- Origin: Italian
- First Use: Medieval times
- Meaning: "Mine" or "Bitter"
- Characteristics: Mia's are often perceived as independent, strong-willed, and possessing a free-spirited nature. They may have a love for adventure.

67. Michelle:
- Origin: French
- First Use: 20th century
- Meaning: "Who is like God?" or "Gift from God"
- Characteristics: Michelles are often associated with grace, elegance, and a refined taste. They may possess a sophisticated and creative nature.

68. Mila:
- Origin: Slavic
- First Use: Medieval times
- Meaning: "Gracious" or "Dear one"
- Characteristics: Milas are often perceived as gentle, kind-hearted, and possessing a warm demeanour. They may have a nurturing and caring nature.

69. Naomi:
- Origin: Hebrew
- First Use: Ancient times
- Meaning: "Pleasant" or "Sweetness"

- Characteristics: Naomis are often associated with sweetness, kindness, and a warm-hearted nature. They may possess a strong sense of empathy.

70. Natalia:
- Origin: Latin
- First Use: Medieval times
- Meaning: "Christmas Day" or "Birthday of the Lord"
- Characteristics: Natalias are often perceived as graceful, elegant, and possessing a refined taste. They may have a love for celebrations and festivities.

71. Natalie:
- Origin: French
- First Use: Medieval times
- Meaning: "Christmas Day" or "Birthday of the Lord"
- Characteristics: Natalies are often associated with warmth, joy, and a friendly demeanour. They may possess a love for social interactions.

72. Nora:
- Origin: Irish
- First Use: 19th century
- Meaning: "Light" or "Honourable"
- Characteristics: Noras are often perceived as gentle, kind-hearted, and possessing a warm demeanour. They may have a calm and composed nature.

73. Nova:
- Origin: Latin
- First Use: 19th century
- Meaning: "New" or "Star"
- Characteristics: Novas are often associated with uniqueness, brightness, and a love for exploration. They may possess a free-spirited and adventurous nature.

74. Olive:
- Origin: Latin

- First Use: Medieval times
- Meaning: "Olive tree" or "Symbol of peace"
- Characteristics: Olives are often perceived as peaceful, wise, and possessing a calm demeanour. They may have a love for harmony and balance.

75. Olivia:
- Origin: Latin
- First Use: Medieval times
- Meaning: "Olive tree" or "Symbol of peace"
- Characteristics: Olivia's are often associated with elegance, grace, and a refined taste. They may possess a sophisticated and creative nature.

76. Paige:
- Origin: English
- First Use: 20th century
- Meaning: "Page" or "Servant"
- Characteristics: Paige's are often perceived as independent, confident, and possessing a strong sense of responsibility. They may have a determined and focused nature.

77. Paisley:
- Origin: Scottish
- First Use: 20th century
- Meaning: "Patterned fabric" or "Church"
- Characteristics: Paisleys are often associated with creativity, uniqueness, and a love for aesthetics. They may possess a free-spirited and artistic nature.

78. Paris:
- Origin: Greek
- First Use: Medieval times
- Meaning: "City of Paris" or "Crafty"
- Characteristics: Parises are often perceived as sophisticated, stylish, and possessing a refined taste. They may have a love for culture and art.

79. Penelope:
- Origin: Greek
- First Use: Ancient times
- Meaning: "Weaver" or "Faithful wife"
- Characteristics: Penelope's are often associated with intelligence, loyalty, and a strong sense of independence. They may possess a determined and resourceful nature.

80. Piper:
- Origin: English
- First Use: 20th century
- Meaning: "Flute player" or "Pipe player"
- Characteristics: Pipers are often perceived as lively, cheerful, and possessing a playful nature. They may have a love for music and entertainment.

81. Quinn:
- Origin: Irish
- First Use: 20th century
- Meaning: "Wisdom" or "Chief leader"
- Characteristics: Quinns are often associated with intelligence, leadership, and a strong sense of fairness. They may possess a diplomatic and determined nature.

82. Raelynn:
- Origin: American
- First Use: 21st century
- Meaning: "Ewe" or "Beautiful lamb"
- Characteristics: Raelynn's are often perceived as gentle, nurturing, and possessing a warm-hearted nature. They may have a love for compassion and kindness.

83. Reese:
- Origin: Welsh
- First Use: 20th century
- Meaning: "Enthusiastic" or "Ardour"

- Characteristics: Reese's are often associated with enthusiasm, energy, and a friendly demeanour. They may possess a social and outgoing nature.

84. Rowan:
- Origin: Gaelic
- First Use: Medieval times
- Meaning: "Little redhead" or "Reddish-brown hair"
- Characteristics: Rowans are often associated with strength, wisdom, and a connection to nature. They may possess a calm and composed demeanour.

85. Ruby:
- Origin: Latin
- First Use: Medieval times
- Meaning: "Red gemstone" or "Deep red colour"
- Characteristics: Rubys are often perceived as passionate, energetic, and possessing a vibrant personality. They may have a love for creativity and self-expression.

86. Rylee:
- Origin: Irish
- First Use: 21st century
- Meaning: "Courageous" or "Valiant"
- Characteristics: Rylee's are often associated with determination, courage, and a strong sense of independence. They may possess a love for challenges and adventure.

87. Sabrina:
- Origin: Celtic
- First Use: Medieval times
- Meaning: "Princess" or "From the border"
- Characteristics: Sabrinas are often perceived as elegant, charming, and possessing a regal demeanour. They may have a refined taste and a love for sophistication.

88. Savannah:
- Origin: Spanish
- First Use: 19th century
- Meaning: "Flat tropical grassland" or "Treeless plain"
- Characteristics: Savannahs are often associated with a free-spirited nature, adaptability, and a love for open spaces. They may possess a warm and friendly demeanour.

89. Scarlett:
- Origin: English
- First Use: Medieval times
- Meaning: "Red" or "Bright red colour"
- Characteristics: Scarlett's are often perceived as passionate, confident, and possessing a bold personality. They may have a love for creativity and self-expression.

90. Seraphina:
- Origin: Hebrew
- First Use: Medieval times
- Meaning: "Fiery" or "Burning one"
- Characteristics: Seraphina's are often associated with warmth, kindness, and a gentle demeanour. They may possess a nurturing and caring nature.

91. Serenity:
- Origin: English
- First Use: 20th century
- Meaning: "Peaceful" or "Tranquil"
- Characteristics: Serenities are often perceived as calm, serene, and possessing a gentle nature. They may have a love for harmony and balance.

92. Skylar:
- Origin: Dutch
- First Use: 20th century
- Meaning: "Scholar" or "Clever one"

- Characteristics: Skylar's are often associated with intelligence, curiosity, and a love for learning. They may possess a friendly and sociable nature.

93. Sofia (and Sophia):
 - Origin: Greek
 - First Use: Medieval times
 - Meaning: "Wisdom" or "Clever"
 - Characteristics: Sofias are often perceived as wise, intelligent, and possessing a warm-hearted nature. They may have a love for knowledge and empathy.

94. Stella:
- Origin: Latin
- First Use: Medieval times
- Meaning: "Star" or "Celestial"
- Characteristics: Stella's are often associated with brightness, charm, and a lively personality. They may possess a love for creativity and self-expression.

95. Trinity:
- Origin: Latin
- First Use: 20th century
- Meaning: "Threefold" or "Triple"
- Characteristics: Trinities are often associated with unity, spirituality, and a balanced nature. They may possess a calm and composed demeanour.

96. Valentina:
- Origin: Latin
- First Use: Medieval times
- Meaning: "Strong" or "Healthy"
- Characteristics: Valentina's are often perceived as strong, determined, and possessing a warm-hearted nature. They may have a love for compassion and kindness.

97. Violet:
- Origin: Latin
- First Use: Medieval times
- Meaning: "Purple" or "Modest"
- Characteristics: Violets are often associated with modesty, elegance, and a refined taste. They may possess a creative and artistic nature.

98. Vivian:
- Origin: Latin
- First Use: Medieval times
- Meaning: "Alive" or "Full of life"
- Characteristics: Vivians are often perceived as vibrant, energetic, and possessing a lively personality. They may have a love for social interactions and a positive outlook on life.

99. Willow:
- Origin: English
- First Use: 20th century
- Meaning: "Graceful" or "Slender"
- Characteristics: Willows are often associated with grace, flexibility, and a love for nature. They may possess a calm and nurturing nature.

100. Zara:
- Origin: Arabic
- First Use: 20th century
- Meaning: "Princess" or "Flower"
- Characteristics: Zaras are often perceived as elegant, graceful, and possessing a regal demeanour. They may have a refined taste and a love for sophistication.

101. Zoe (and Zoey):
- Origin: Greek
- First Use: Ancient times
- Meaning: "Life" or "Alive"
- Characteristics: Zoes are often associated with vitality, positivity, and a love for life. They may possess a friendly and optimistic nature.

Gender-Neutral Names

1. Addison:
- Origin: English
- First Use: 17th century
- Meaning: "Son of Adam" or "son of the red earth"
- Characteristics: Addison is a unisex name often associated with individuals who are creative, communicative, and have a friendly disposition.

2. Aidley:
- Origin: English
- First Use: Modern creation
- Meaning: Derived from Aiden, meaning "little fire" or "fiery one"
- Characteristics: Aidley may be associated with warmth, energy, and a lively personality.

3. Ainsley:
- Origin: Scottish
- First Use: Medieval times
- Meaning: "One's own meadow" or "woodland clearing"
- Characteristics: Ainsley is often associated with individuals who are harmonious, nature-loving, and possess a sense of peace.

4. Alex:
- Origin: Greek
- First Use: Ancient times
- Meaning: "Defender of the people"

- Characteristics: A versatile and widely used name, Alex can be associated with individuals who are adaptable, sociable, and exhibit leadership qualities.

5. Ali:
- Origin: Arabic
- First Use: Ancient times
- Meaning: "Exalted" or "sublime"
- Characteristics: Ali is a name often associated with individuals who are noble, honorable, and possess a strong sense of integrity.

6. Amory:
- Origin: Germanic
- First Use: Medieval times
- Meaning: "Brave" or "powerful"
- Characteristics: Amory is a name associated with strength, courage, and resilience. Individuals with this name may be seen as determined and assertive.

7. Andie:
- Origin: Greek
- First Use: Modern variation of Andrew
- Meaning: "Manly" or "brave"
- Characteristics: Andie is often associated with individuals who are courageous, strong-willed, and possess a sense of adventure.

8. Archer:
- Origin: English
- First Use: Medieval times
- Meaning: "Bowman" or "one who uses a bow and arrow"
- Characteristics: Archer is a name associated with precision, focus, and determination. It may be linked to individuals who are goal-oriented and ambitious.

9. Arden:
- Origin: English
- First Use: Medieval times

- Meaning: "Eagle valley" or "eagle's den"
- Characteristics: Arden is often associated with individuals who are free-spirited, independent, and have a love for nature.

10. Ari:
- Origin: Hebrew
- First Use: Ancient times
- Meaning: "Lion" or "eagle"
- Characteristics: Ari is a name associated with strength, courage, and leadership. Individuals with this name may be perceived as bold and confident.

11. Armani:
- Origin: Italian
- First Use: Modern creation
- Meaning: Derived from the Italian fashion brand
- Characteristics: Armani is a name associated with style, sophistication, and elegance. Individuals with this name may have a keen sense of aesthetics.

12. Ash:
- Origin: English
- First Use: Medieval times
- Meaning: "Ash tree"
- Characteristics: Ash is often associated with individuals who are grounded, practical, and possess a calm and stable demeanour.

13. Aspen:
- Origin: English
- First Use: Modern nature-inspired name
- Meaning: "Aspen tree"
- Characteristics: Aspen is associated with individuals who appreciate nature, are adaptable, and may have a serene disposition.

14. Atlas:
- Origin: Greek
- First Use: Ancient times

- Meaning: "Bearer of the heavens" or "enduring"
- Characteristics: Atlas is a name associated with strength, endurance, and a sense of responsibility. Individuals with this name may be perceived as reliable and capable.

15. Bailey:
- Origin: English
- First Use: Medieval times
- Meaning: "Bailiff" or "steward"
- Characteristics: Bailey is often associated with individuals who are responsible, organized, and may have a natural leadership ability.

16. Baker:
- Origin: English
- First Use: Occupational surname
- Meaning: "Baker"
- Characteristics: Baker is a name associated with individuals who may have a passion for culinary arts, hard work, and attention to detail.

17. Bay:
- Origin: English
- First Use: Modern nature-inspired name
- Meaning: "Inlet" or "small body of water"
- Characteristics: Bay is often associated with individuals who appreciate nature, are calm, and possess a sense of tranquillity.

18. Bellamy:
- Origin: French
- First Use: Medieval times
- Meaning: "Beautiful friend"
- Characteristics: Bellamy is often associated with individuals who are sociable, charming, and have a friendly and approachable demeanour.

19. Billy:
- Origin: English
- First Use: Medieval times (as a diminutive of William)
- Meaning: "Resolute protector"

- Characteristics: Billy is often associated with individuals who are determined, loyal, and possess a strong sense of protection.

20. Blair:
- Origin: Scottish
- First Use: Medieval times
- Meaning: "Field" or "plain"
- Characteristics: Blair is often associated with individuals who are serene, down-to-earth, and have a calm and composed demeanour.

21. Blake:
- Origin: Old English
- First Use: Medieval times
- Meaning: "Black" or "pale"
- Characteristics: Blake is often associated with individuals who are strong-willed, confident, and may have a mysterious or enigmatic quality.

22. Blue:
- Origin: English (Colour as a Name)
- First Use: Modern nature-inspired name
- Meaning: The colour blue
- Characteristics: Blue is a unique and modern name associated with qualities such as calmness, tranquillity, and creativity.

23. Bobby:
- Origin: English (Diminutive of Robert)
- First Use: Medieval times
- Meaning: "Bright fame"
- Characteristics: Bobby is often associated with individuals who are friendly, approachable, and have a down-to-earth personality.

24. Brady:
- Origin: Irish
- First Use: Medieval times
- Meaning: "Broad eye" or "spirited"

- Characteristics: Brady is a name associated with individuals who are lively, energetic, and may have a cheerful disposition.

25. Brighton:
- Origin: English
- First Use: Modern creation
- Meaning: "Bright town" or "beautiful city"
- Characteristics: Brighton is often associated with individuals who appreciate beauty, are sociable, and may have a positive and optimistic outlook.

26. Brooke:
- Origin: English
- First Use: Medieval times
- Meaning: "Small stream" or "brook"
- Characteristics: Brooke is a name associated with individuals who are calm, nurturing, and possess a gentle and kind-hearted nature.

27. Carroll:
- Origin: Irish
- First Use: Medieval times
- Meaning: "Champion" or "warrior"
- Characteristics: Carroll is often associated with individuals who are strong-willed, determined, and may exhibit leadership qualities.

28. Casey:
- Origin: Irish
- First Use: Medieval times
- Meaning: "Descendant of Cathasaigh" or "vigilant"
- Characteristics: Casey is a name associated with individuals who are watchful, alert, and may have a protective nature.

29. Channing:
- Origin: English
- First Use: Medieval times
- Meaning: "Young wolf" or "official of the church"

- Characteristics: Channing is often associated with individuals who are confident, independent, and may possess a strong sense of individuality.

30. Charley:
- Origin: Germanic
- First Use: Medieval times
- Meaning: "Free man" or "strong"
- Characteristics: Charley is a name associated with individuals who value freedom, independence, and may have a spirited and adventurous personality.

31. Clay:
- Origin: Old English
- First Use: Medieval times
- Meaning: "Mud" or "earth"
- Characteristics: Clay is often associated with individuals who are grounded, practical, and may have a strong connection to nature.

32. Corey:
- Origin: Irish
- First Use: Medieval times
- Meaning: "Hollow" or "dweller in or near a hollow"
- Characteristics: Corey is a name associated with individuals who are introspective, adaptable, and may have a calm and composed demeanour.

33. Dakota:
- Origin: Native American (Sioux)
- First Use: Modern nature-inspired name
- Meaning: "Friend" or "ally"
- Characteristics: Dakota is often associated with individuals who are friendly, sociable, and may have a strong sense of camaraderie.

34. Dallas:
- Origin: Scottish
- First Use: Medieval times
- Meaning: "Meadow dwelling"

- Characteristics: Dallas is a name associated with individuals who are sociable, outgoing, and may have a friendly and approachable nature.

35. Dawson:
- Origin: English
- First Use: Medieval times
- Meaning: "Son of David" or "beloved"
- Characteristics: Dawson is often associated with individuals who are beloved, caring, and may have a nurturing personality.

36. Denver:
- Origin: English
- First Use: Modern nature-inspired name
- Meaning: "Green valley" or "from Anvers"
- Characteristics: Denver is associated with individuals who appreciate nature, are down-to-earth, and may have a calm and composed demeanour.

37. Drew:
- Origin: Old English
- First Use: Medieval times
- Meaning: "Wisdom" or "courage"
- Characteristics: Drew is a name associated with individuals who are wise, courageous, and may have a strong sense of justice.

38. Dru:
- Origin: French
- First Use: Medieval times
- Meaning: Variant of Drew, meaning "wise" or "courageous"
- Characteristics: Dru shares characteristics with Drew, being associated with wisdom, courage, and a sense of justice.

39. Ellison:
- Origin: English
- First Use: Medieval times
- Meaning: "Son of Ellis" or "Jehovah is God"

- Characteristics: Ellison is often associated with individuals who are strong-willed, determined, and may have a leadership mindset.

40. Emerson:
- Origin: English
- First Use: Medieval times
- Meaning: "Son of Emery" or "bravery"
- Characteristics: Emerson is a name associated with bravery, resilience, and may be linked to individuals with a strong sense of integrity.

41. Florian:
- Origin: Latin
- First Use: Ancient times
- Meaning: "Flower" or "blooming"
- Characteristics: Florian is often associated with individuals who are artistic, sensitive, and have a gentle and refined nature.

42. Frankie:
- Origin: English
- First Use: 19th century
- Meaning: "Free one" or "from France"
- Characteristics: Frankie is often associated with individuals who are free-spirited, independent, and may have a playful and lively personality.

43. Gene:
- Origin: Greek
- First Use: 19th century
- Meaning: "Well-born" or "noble"
- Characteristics: Gene is a name associated with individuals who may have refined manners, a sense of dignity, and noble qualities.

44. Hadley:
- Origin: English
- First Use: Medieval times
- Meaning: "Heath covered meadow" or "field of heather"

- Characteristics: Hadley is often associated with individuals who appreciate nature, are down-to-earth, and may have a calm and composed demeanour.

45. Harley:
- Origin: English
- First Use: Medieval times
- Meaning: "Hare's meadow" or "rock meadow"
- Characteristics: Harley is a name associated with individuals who may have a strong and energetic personality, as well as a love for adventure.

46. Harper:
- Origin: English
- First Use: Medieval times (as a surname)
- Meaning: "Harp player" or "minstrel"
- Characteristics: Harper is often associated with individuals who are creative, musical, and may have a poetic and artistic nature.

47. Hayden:
- Origin: English
- First Use: Medieval times
- Meaning: "Valley of hay" or "heathen"
- Characteristics: Hayden is a name associated with individuals who are grounded, practical, and may have a calm and steady demeanour.

48. Indigo:
- Origin: English (Colour as a Name)
- First Use: Modern nature-inspired name
- Meaning: The colour indigo
- Characteristics: Indigo is a unique and modern name associated with qualities such as creativity, intuition, and a free-spirited nature.

49. Jaden:
- Origin: Modern creation
- First Use: Late 20th century
- Meaning: A modern name with various interpretations, often associated with a combination of names or invented meanings.

- Characteristics: Jaden is often associated with individuals who are modern, innovative, and may have a dynamic and progressive mindset.

50. Jagger:
- Origin: English
- First Use: Modern creation
- Meaning: "Carter" or "peddler"
- Characteristics: Jagger is often associated with individuals who are energetic, charismatic, and may have a bold and adventurous personality.

51. Jamie:
- Origin: English
- First Use: Medieval times (as a nickname for James)
- Meaning: "Supplanter" or "one who follows"
- Characteristics: Jamie is often associated with individuals who are adaptable, friendly, and may have a sociable and easy-going nature.

52. Jan:
- Origin: Dutch
- First Use: Medieval times (as a diminutive of John)
- Meaning: "God is gracious"
- Characteristics: Jan is often associated with individuals who are gracious, kind-hearted, and may have a strong sense of compassion.

53. Jayden:
- Origin: Modern creation
- First Use: Late 20th century
- Meaning: A modern name with various interpretations, often associated with a combination of names or invented meanings.
- Characteristics: Jayden is often associated with individuals who are modern, innovative, and may have a dynamic and progressive mindset.

54. Jean:
- Origin: French
- First Use: Medieval times (as a diminutive of John)
- Meaning: "God is gracious"

- Characteristics: Jean is often associated with individuals who are gracious, refined, and may have a sophisticated and elegant nature.

55. Jericho:
- Origin: Hebrew
- First Use: Ancient times
- Meaning: "City of the moon" or "fragrant"
- Characteristics: Jericho is often associated with individuals who are resilient, determined, and may have a strong sense of endurance.

56. Jody:
- Origin: English
- First Use: Modern times
- Meaning: "Jehovah's gift"
- Characteristics: Jody is often associated with individuals who are generous, caring, and may have a nurturing personality.

57. Jude:
- Origin: Hebrew
- First Use: Ancient times
- Meaning: "Praise" or "thanks"
- Characteristics: Jude is often associated with individuals who are grateful, humble, and may have a strong sense of appreciation for life.

58. Kelly:
- Origin: Irish
- First Use: Medieval times
- Meaning: "Bright-headed" or "warrior"
- Characteristics: Kelly is a name associated with individuals who are strong-willed, confident, and may have a warrior spirit.

59. Kit:
- Origin: Greek
- First Use: Medieval times (as a diminutive of Christopher)
- Meaning: "Bearer of Christ" or "Christ-bearer"
- Characteristics: Kit is often associated with individuals who are compassionate, kind-hearted, and may have a nurturing nature.

60. Layton:
- Origin: English
- First Use: Medieval times
- Meaning: "Settlement with a leek garden" or "meadow town"
- Characteristics: Layton is often associated with individuals who are practical, down-to-earth, and may have a calm and composed demeanour.

61. Lennon:
- Origin: Irish
- First Use: Modern times
- Meaning: "Lover" or "dear one"
- Characteristics: Lennon is often associated with individuals who are artistic, free-spirited, and may have a love for music or creativity.

62. Leslie:
- Origin: Scottish
- First Use: Medieval times (as a surname)
- Meaning: "Garden of holly" or "gray fortress"
- Characteristics: Leslie is often associated with individuals who are versatile, adaptable, and may have a calm and collected nature.

63. Lindsay:
- Origin: Scottish
- First Use: Medieval times (as a surname)
- Meaning: "Lincoln's island" or "lake settlement"
- Characteristics: Lindsay is often associated with individuals who are sociable, outgoing, and may have a friendly and approachable demeanour.

64. Lou:
- Origin: Germanic
- First Use: Medieval times (as a diminutive of Louis)
- Meaning: "Famous warrior" or "renowned in battle"
- Characteristics: Lou is often associated with individuals who are courageous, strong-willed, and may have a determined and assertive nature.

65. Maddox:
- Origin: Welsh
- First Use: Medieval times (as a surname)
- Meaning: "Son of Madoc" or "fortunate"
- Characteristics: Maddox is often associated with individuals who are adventurous, bold, and may have a charismatic and dynamic personality.

66. Marley:
- Origin: English
- First Use: Modern times
- Meaning: "Meadow near the lake" or "pleasant wood"
- Characteristics: Marley is often associated with individuals who are laid-back, nature-loving, and may have a peaceful and easy-going nature.

67. Maxwell:
- Origin: Scottish
- First Use: Medieval times (as a surname)
- Meaning: "Mack's spring" or "great stream"
- Characteristics: Maxwell is often associated with individuals who are confident, ambitious, and may have a strong and determined personality.

68. Micah:
- Origin: Hebrew
- First Use: Ancient times
- Meaning: "Who is like God?"
- Characteristics: Micah is often associated with individuals who are compassionate, humble, and may have a strong sense of justice.

69. Milan:
- Origin: Slavic
- First Use: Ancient times
- Meaning: "Gracious" or "dear"

- Characteristics: Milan is often associated with individuals who are elegant, refined, and may have a sophisticated and cultured nature.

70. Miller:
- Origin: English
- First Use: Medieval times (as an occupational surname)
- Meaning: "Grain grinder" or "miller"
- Characteristics: Miller is often associated with individuals who are hardworking, practical, and may have a strong work ethic.

71. Morgan:
- Origin: Welsh
- First Use: Medieval times (as a surname)
- Meaning: "Sea-born" or "bright circle"
- Characteristics: Morgan is often associated with individuals who are independent, adaptable, and may have a strong sense of individuality.

72. Nevada:
- Origin: Spanish
- First Use: Modern times
- Meaning: "Snowy" or "covered in snow"
- Characteristics: Nevada is often associated with individuals who appreciate nature, may have a calm and serene disposition, and a love for winter landscapes.

73. Pascalle:
- Origin: French
- First Use: Medieval times
- Meaning: "Easter child" or "born on Easter"
- Characteristics: Pascalle is often associated with individuals who are gentle, nurturing, and may have a caring and compassionate nature.

74. Pat:
- Origin: English (Diminutive of Patrick)
- First Use: Medieval times
- Meaning: "Noble" or "nobleman"

- Characteristics: Pat is often associated with individuals who are dignified, honourable, and may have a strong sense of integrity.

75. Puma:
- Origin: Quechuan (Indigenous South American)
- First Use: Modern times
- Meaning: Refers to a large cat species
- Characteristics: Puma is often associated with individuals who are fierce, independent, and may have a strong and assertive personality.

76. Quincy:
- Origin: Latin
- First Use: Medieval times (as a surname)
- Meaning: "Fifth son" or "estate of the fifth son"
- Characteristics: Quincy is often associated with individuals who are charismatic, sociable, and may have a friendly and approachable nature.

77. Raleigh:
- Origin: Old English
- First Use: Medieval times (as a surname)
- Meaning: "Red clearing" or "roe deer clearing"
- Characteristics: Raleigh is often associated with individuals who are determined, bold, and may have a dynamic and adventurous personality.

78. Ramsey:
- Origin: Old English
- First Use: Medieval times (as a surname)
- Meaning: "Wild garlic island" or "island of rams"
- Characteristics: Ramsey is often associated with individuals who are practical, grounded, and may have a strong connection to nature.

79. Ray:
- Origin: Germanic
- First Use: Medieval times (as a short form of Raymond)
- Meaning: "Counsel" or "protector"

- Characteristics: Ray is often associated with individuals who are protective, wise, and may have a nurturing nature.

80. Rayne:
- Origin: English
- First Use: Modern times
- Meaning: "Counsel" or "mighty"
- Characteristics: Rayne is often associated with individuals who are strong-willed, independent, and may have a powerful and resilient personality.

81. Riley:
- Origin: Irish
- First Use: Medieval times (as a surname)
- Meaning: "Valiant" or "courageous"
- Characteristics: Riley is often associated with individuals who are spirited, energetic, and may possess a sense of adventure.

82. Rio:
- Origin: Spanish/Portuguese
- First Use: Modern times
- Meaning: "River" or "stream"
- Characteristics: Rio is often associated with individuals who are free-spirited, fluid, and may have a lively and dynamic personality.

83. Ripley:
- Origin: Old English
- First Use: Medieval times (as a surname)
- Meaning: "Strip of clearing" or "hrypa's meadow"
- Characteristics: Ripley is often associated with individuals who are independent, determined, and may have a strong connection to nature.

84. River:
- Origin: English
- First Use: Modern times (as a nature-inspired name)
- Meaning: "Body of water flowing towards the sea"

- Characteristics: River is often associated with individuals who appreciate nature, are calm, and may have a serene disposition.

85. Remi:
- Origin: French
- First Use: Medieval times
- Meaning: "Oarsman" or "remedy"
- Characteristics: Remi is often associated with individuals who are adaptable, resourceful, and may have a healing or comforting presence.

86. Sam:
- Origin: Hebrew
- First Use: Medieval times (as a short form of Samuel)
- Meaning: "Heard by God"
- Characteristics: Sam is often associated with individuals who are approachable, friendly, and may have a warm and caring nature.

87. Sasha:
- Origin: Russian
- First Use: Modern times
- Meaning: "Defender of mankind"
- Characteristics: Sasha is often associated with individuals who are protective, compassionate, and may have a strong sense of justice.

88. Sawyer:
- Origin: Middle English
- First Use: Medieval times (as an occupational surname)
- Meaning: "Woodcutter" or "one who saws wood"
- Characteristics: Sawyer is often associated with individuals who are industrious, practical, and may have a strong work ethic.

89. Sidney:
- Origin: Old English
- First Use: Medieval times (as a surname)
- Meaning: "Wide island" or "wide meadow"

- Characteristics: Sidney is often associated with individuals who are sociable, adaptable, and may have a friendly and approachable demeanour.

90. Spencer:
- Origin: Old French
- First Use: Medieval times (as an occupational surname)
- Meaning: "Steward" or "dispenser of provisions"
- Characteristics: Spencer is often associated with individuals who are responsible, organized, and may have a natural leadership ability.

91. Sunny:
- Origin: English
- First Use: Modern times (as a nature-inspired name)
- Meaning: "Bright" or "radiant"
- Characteristics: Sunny is often associated with individuals who have a cheerful, optimistic disposition and bring warmth to those around them.

92. Sydney:
- Origin: Old English
- First Use: Medieval times (as a surname)
- Meaning: "Wide island" or "wide meadow"
- Characteristics: Sydney shares characteristics with Sidney and is often associated with sociable, adaptable individuals with a friendly nature.

93. Taylor:
- Origin: Old French
- First Use: Medieval times (as an occupational surname)
- Meaning: "Tailor" or "cutter of cloth"
- Characteristics: Taylor is often associated with individuals who are creative, detail-oriented, and may have a keen sense of fashion.

94. Teagan:
- Origin: Irish
- First Use: Modern times
- Meaning: "Little poet" or "attractive"

- Characteristics: Teagan is often associated with individuals who are creative, poetic, and may have a charming and attractive personality.

95. Tesla:
- Origin: Slavic
- First Use: Modern times
- Meaning: Derived from the surname of inventor Nikola Tesla
- Characteristics: Tesla is often associated with individuals who are innovative, curious, and may have a strong interest in science and technology.

96. Theo:
- Origin: Greek
- First Use: Ancient times
- Meaning: "God" or "divine"
- Characteristics: Theo is often associated with individuals who are compassionate, wise, and may have a spiritual or philosophical nature.

97. Tobin:
- Origin: Irish
- First Use: Medieval times (as a surname)
- Meaning: "From the house of Tobias" or "God is good"
- Characteristics: Tobin is often associated with individuals who are kind-hearted, dependable, and may have a strong sense of goodness.

98. Toshi:
- Origin: Japanese
- First Use: Modern times
- Meaning: "Alert" or "wise"
- Characteristics: Toshi is often associated with individuals who are perceptive, wise, and may have a calm and composed demeanour.

99. Tyler:
- Origin: Old English
- First Use: Medieval times (as a surname)
- Meaning: "Tile maker" or "roof builder"

- Characteristics: Tyler is often associated with individuals who are hardworking, practical, and may have a strong sense of craftsmanship.

100.   Walker:
- Origin: Old English
- First Use: Medieval times (as an occupational surname)
- Meaning: "Cloth-walker" or "fuller of cloth"
- Characteristics: Walker is often associated with individuals who are industrious, determined, and may have a strong work ethic.

101.   Wilder:
- Origin: English
- First Use: Modern times
- Meaning: "Untamed" or "wild"
- Characteristics: Wilder is often associated with individuals who are adventurous, free-spirited, and may have a bold and dynamic personality.

Unusual Names

1. Alaric:
- Origin: Germanic.
- First Use: Historically used by the Visigoths, notably borne by the King of the Visigoths who sacked Rome in 410 AD.
- Meaning: "Ruler of All" or "Ruler of All People".

2. Althaea:
- Origin: Greek.
- First Use: In Greek mythology, Althaea was the mother of Meleager.
- Meaning: Possibly derived from Greek "althaino", meaning "to heal". Associated with the marshmallow plant.

3. Althea:
- Origin: Greek.
- First Use: Ancient Greece.
- Meaning: "Healing" or "Wholesome". Associated with nurturing and healing in Greek mythology.

4. Amadis:
- Origin: Derived from Latin "Amatus", meaning "beloved".
- First Use: Medieval literature, particularly in Arthurian and chivalric romances.
- Meaning: "Beloved" or "Loved One".

5. Amaryllis:
- Origin: Greek.
- First Use: Associated with Greek pastoral poetry.

- Meaning: "To sparkle" or "Fresh". Commonly used as a flower name.

6. Apollonia:
- Origin: Greek.
- First Use: Ancient Greece.
- Meaning: Dedicated to Apollo, the Greek god of music and arts.

7. Aurelius:
- Origin: Latin.
- First Use: Ancient Rome.
- Meaning: "Golden" or "Gilded". Common Roman family name.

8. Avalon:
- Origin: Celtic.
- First Use: Arthurian legend, associated with the mythical island of Avalon.
- Meaning: Unclear, often associated with paradise or apple orchards.

9. Azalea:
- Origin: Greek.
- First Use: The name of the flowering shrub.
- Meaning: "Dry" or "Arid", metaphorically associated with the flower.

10. Azura:
- Origin: Persian.
- First Use: Modern name.
- Meaning: "Sky Blue" or "Clear Blue Sky".

11. Balthasar:
- Origin: Babylonian/Persian.
- First Use: Biblical, associated with one of the Magi.
- Meaning: "Baal protect the king".

12. Basil:
- Origin: Greek.
- First Use: Ancient Greece.

- Meaning: "Royal" or "Kingly". Also associated with the herb basil, symbolizing good wishes.

13. Belphoebe:
- Origin: Created by Edmund Spenser.
- First Use: In Spenser's "The Faerie Queene" (16th century).
- Meaning: The name was coined by Spenser and doesn't have a clear historical meaning. Represents the idea of "beautiful light".

14. Briseis:
- Origin: Greek.
- First Use: In Greek mythology, where Briseis was a Trojan woman captured by Achilles during the Trojan War.
- Meaning: Possibly derived from the Greek word "bris", meaning "to be strong" or "to be forceful".

15. Caius:
- Origin: Latin.
- First Use: Ancient Rome.
- Meaning: Possibly derived from the Latin word "gaius", meaning "happy" or "rejoice". Common Roman given name.

16. Calista:
- Origin: Greek.
- First Use: Ancient Greece.
- Meaning: "Most beautiful" or "Very Beautiful".

17. Calliope:
- Origin: Greek.
- First Use: In Greek mythology, Calliope is the muse of epic poetry.
- Meaning: "Beautiful Voice" or "Beautifully Voiced".

18. Calypso:
- Origin: Greek.
- First Use: In Greek mythology, Calypso is a nymph who detains Odysseus on her island.
- Meaning: "Concealer" or "She who hides".

19. Caspian:
- Origin: Derived from the Caspian Sea.
- First Use: Popularized by C.S. Lewis in "The Chronicles of Narnia".
- Meaning: Associated with the Caspian Sea region.

20. Cerys:
- Origin: Welsh.
- First Use: Modern name.
- Meaning: "Love" or "To love".

21. Cleon:
- Origin: Greek.
- First Use: Ancient Greece.
- Meaning: "Proud", "Famous", or "Renowned".

22. Cyprian:
- Origin: Greek.
- First Use: Ancient Greece.
- Meaning: "From Cyprus". Also associated with the word "cypress", a type of tree.

23. Damaris:
- Origin: Greek.
- First Use: Mentioned in the New Testament in the Bible (Acts 17:34).
- Meaning: Likely derived from the Greek word "damalis", meaning "calf" or "heifer".

24. Daxton:
- Origin: Modern, possibly American.
- First Use: Modern name.
- Meaning: No widely recognized historical meaning; likely a contemporary invented name.

25. Dorian:
- Origin: Greek.
- First Use: Ancient Greece.
- Meaning: "Of Doris" or "Gift".

26. Drystan:
- Origin: Welsh.
- First Use: In Welsh mythology and Arthurian legend.
- Meaning: Possibly derived from the Welsh word "trystan", meaning "tumult" or "riot".

27. Eirian:
- Origin: Welsh.
- First Use: Welsh name.
- Meaning: "Bright", "Beautiful", or "Radiant".

28. Eirlys:
- Origin: Welsh.
- First Use: Welsh name.
- Meaning: "Snowdrop" or "Snowflake".

29. Elara:
- Origin: Greek.
- First Use: In Greek mythology, Elara was a moon of Jupiter.
- Meaning: Possibly derived from Greek "elairo", meaning "to shine".

30. Elestren:
- Origin: Cornish.
- First Use: Cornish name.
- Meaning: "Illumination" or "Beautiful".

31. Elowen:
- Origin: Cornish.
- First Use: Cornish name.
- Meaning: "Elm Tree".

32. Elysia:
- Origin: Greek.
- First Use: Modern name.
- Meaning: "Blissful" or "Of Elysium" (Elysium being a place of ideal happiness in Greek mythology).

33. Endymion:
- Origin: Greek.
- First Use: In Greek mythology, Endymion was a handsome shepherd loved by the moon goddess Selene.
- Meaning: Uncertain, possibly "Diver" or "Plunger".

34. Eudoxia:
- Origin: Greek.
- First Use: Ancient Greece.
- Meaning: "Good Glory" or "Favoured by Good Fortune".

35. Eulalia:
- Origin: Greek.
- First Use: Ancient Greece.
- Meaning: "Sweetly Speaking" or "Well-spoken".

36. Eulalie:
- Origin: Greek.
- First Use: Ancient Greece.
- Meaning: "Sweetly Speaking" or "Well-spoken". Similar to Eulalia.

37. Evadne:
- Origin: Greek.
- First Use: In Greek mythology, Evadne was the wife of Capaneus.
- Meaning: "Pleasing" or "Gracious".

38. Faelan:
- Origin: Irish/Gaelic.
- First Use: Gaelic name.
- Meaning: "Little Wolf".

39. Faeryn:
- Origin: Modern, likely invented.
- First Use: Modern name.
- Meaning: No widely recognized historical meaning; possibly inspired by the word "faery" or "fairy".

40. Finlo:
- Origin: Scottish.
- First Use: Scottish name.
- Meaning: "Fair Hero" or "Fair Warrior".

41. Galadriel:
- Origin: Created by J.R.R. Tolkien for "The Lord of the Rings".
- First Use: In Tolkien's Middle-earth legendarium.
- Meaning: The name is Elvish and is often interpreted as "Maiden crowned with a radiant garland". It carries a sense of beauty and nobility.

42. Gideon:
- Origin: Hebrew.
- First Use: In the Bible (Judges 6-8).
- Meaning: "Feller" or "Hewer", suggesting someone who cuts down trees. In a biblical context, Gideon was a judge and military leader.

43. Gwydion:
- Origin: Welsh.
- First Use: In Welsh mythology.
- Meaning: Possibly derived from the Welsh elements "gwy" meaning "hay" and "dion" meaning "god" or "deity". Gwydion is a powerful magician and hero in Welsh mythology.

44. Hadriel:
- Origin: Combination of Hebrew "Hadassah" and "El".
- First Use: Modern name.
- Meaning: A modern and creative name, combining elements from Hebrew names, possibly meaning "Myrtle of God".

45. Halcyon:
- Origin: Greek.
- First Use: In Greek mythology.
- Meaning: "Kingfisher" or "Calm, peaceful". In mythology, Alcyone (a variant) was transformed into a kingfisher.

46. Helianthe:
- Origin: French, derived from Greek.
- First Use: Modern name.
- Meaning: "Sunflower". A floral name inspired by the sunflower, reflecting warmth and brightness.

47. Icarus:
- Origin: Greek.
- First Use: In Greek mythology.
- Meaning: Derived from the Greek word "íkaros", possibly meaning "follower". Icarus is known for flying too close to the sun with wings of feathers and wax.

48. Ignatius:
- Origin: Latin.
- First Use: Ancient Rome.
- Meaning: "Fiery" or "Fiery One". It was a common Roman given name and later adopted by early Christians.

49. Iliad:
- Origin: Greek.
- First Use: Ancient Greece.
- Meaning: Refers to the epic poem attributed to Homer, detailing events of the Trojan War.

50. Inidara:
- Origin: Modern, likely invented.
- First Use: Modern name.
- Meaning: No widely recognized historical meaning; a creative and unique name.

51. Iolanthe:
- Origin: Greek.
- First Use: In Greek mythology.
- Meaning: "Violet Flower" or "Violet". A name associated with nature and beauty.

52. Isabeau:
- Origin: French.
- First Use: Medieval France.
- Meaning: A variant of Isabel/Isabella, meaning "God is my oath".

53. Isidore:
- Origin: Greek.
- First Use: Ancient Greece.
- Meaning: "Gift of Isis" or "Gift of the goddess". Isis was an Egyptian goddess.

54. Isolabella:
- Origin: Italian.
- First Use: Modern name.
- Meaning: "Beautiful Isolde". A creative combination of "Isolde" (see below) and "bella" meaning "beautiful".

55. Isolde:
- Origin: Celtic.
- First Use: In Arthurian legend.
- Meaning: "Fair" or "Beautiful". Isolde is a tragic heroine in Arthurian romance.

56. Jocasta:
- Origin: Greek.
- First Use: In Greek mythology.
- Meaning: "Shining Moon" or "Bright Star". Jocasta was a queen in Greek mythology.

57. Jocelyn:
- Origin: Germanic.
- First Use: Medieval France.
- Meaning: "Joyous" or "Merry".

58. Jovian:
- Origin: Latin.
- First Use: Ancient Rome.

- Meaning: "Related to Jupiter". Jovian was a Roman Emperor.

59. Kaelith:
- Origin: Modern, likely invented.
- First Use: Modern name.
- Meaning: No widely recognized historical meaning; a creative and unique name.

60. Kairi:
- Origin: Modern, possibly Japanese.
- First Use: Modern name.
- Meaning: While it may have Japanese associations, its specific meaning can depend on cultural interpretations. In Japanese, "kai" can mean "sea", and "ri" can mean "village".

61. Leocadia:
- Origin: Greek.
- First Use: Ancient Greece.
- Meaning: "Bright" or "Clear". It's a name associated with light and clarity.

62. Lirael:
- Origin: Modern, likely invented.
- First Use: Popularized by Garth Nix in his fantasy novels, particularly the "Old Kingdom" series.
- Meaning: The meaning is not widely known. It was created by the author for his fictional work.

63. Lysander:
- Origin: Greek.
- First Use: Ancient Greece.
- Meaning: "Liberator" or "Freeing Men". Lysander was a Spartan military general in ancient Greece.

64. Lysandra:
- Origin: Greek.
- First Use: Ancient Greece.

- Meaning: "Liberator" or "Freeing Men". Similar to Lysander.

65. Morpheus:
- Origin: Greek.
- First Use: In Greek mythology.
- Meaning: "Shape" or "Form". Morpheus is the god of dreams, known for shaping and appearing in dreams.

66. Morvran:
- Origin: Welsh.
- First Use: In Welsh mythology.
- Meaning: Possibly derived from the Welsh elements "mor" meaning "sea" and "bran" meaning "crow" or "raven". Morvran is a legendary figure associated with magic and prophecy.

67. Myrrh:
- Origin: Arabic.
- First Use: Ancient times.
- Meaning: A fragrant resin obtained from certain trees, often used in perfumes and incense.

68. Nereus:
- Origin: Greek.
- First Use: In Greek mythology.
- Meaning: "Wet One" or "Drenched". Nereus is a sea god often described as an old man of the sea.

69. Nyssa:
- Origin: Greek.
- First Use: Ancient Greece.
- Meaning: "Beginning" or "New Beginning".

70. Nyx:
- Origin: Greek.
- First Use: In Greek mythology.
- Meaning: "Night". Nyx is the primordial goddess of the night.

71. Oberon:
- Origin: English/French.
- First Use: In medieval literature, particularly in the legend of "Huon of Bordeaux".
- Meaning: Uncertain, possibly derived from Old Germanic "Alberich" meaning "elf ruler". Oberon is a legendary fairy king.

72. Octavian:
- Origin: Latin.
- First Use: Ancient Rome.
- Meaning: "Eighth". It was a common Roman praenomen. Octavian was the birth name of the Roman Emperor Augustus.

73. Ondine:
- Origin: French.
- First Use: Derived from European folklore.
- Meaning: A water nymph or mermaid, often associated with bodies of water.

74. Orin:
- Origin: Irish.
- First Use: Irish name.
- Meaning: "Dark-haired" or "From the Riverbank".

75. Orion:
- Origin: Greek.
- First Use: In Greek mythology.
- Meaning: Possibly "Rising in the Sky" or "Hunter". Orion was a legendary hunter.

76. Osiris:
- Origin: Egyptian.
- First Use: Ancient Egypt.
- Meaning: Uncertain, possibly "throne" or "seat of the eye". Osiris is a major god in ancient Egyptian religion.

77. Paxton:
- Origin: English.
- First Use: Modern name.
- Meaning: "Peace Town" or "Town of Peace".

78. Persephone:
- Origin: Greek.
- First Use: In Greek mythology.
- Meaning: "Bringer of Destruction" or "Destroyer of Light". Persephone is the queen of the Underworld in Greek mythology.

79. Pyrrha:
- Origin: Greek.
- First Use: In Greek mythology.
- Meaning: "Fiery" or "Red-Haired". Pyrrha was a woman in Greek mythology associated with the flood and the creation of humans.

80. Pyrrhus:
- Origin: Greek.
- First Use: In ancient Greece.
- Meaning: "Red" or "Flame-coloured". Pyrrhus was a king of Epirus in ancient Greece.

81. Quillian:
- Origin: Modern, likely invented.
- First Use: Modern name.
- Meaning: The meaning is not widely known. It appears to be a creative and unique name.

82. Quillon:
- Origin: Latin.
- First Use: Modern name.
- Meaning: Possibly derived from the Latin word "quillonem", meaning "cross-guard" (as in the hilt of a sword).

83. Rhydian:
- Origin: Welsh.

- First Use: Welsh name.
- Meaning: "Ford" or "Watercourse". It's a name associated with rivers and water.

84. Riantha:
- Origin: Modern, likely invented.
- First Use: Modern name.
- Meaning: The meaning is not widely known. It appears to be a creative and unique name.

85. Rowena:
- Origin: Germanic.
- First Use: Used in medieval romance literature.
- Meaning: "Fame" or "Joyful". Rowena is a name with historical and literary significance.

86. Seraphiel:
- Origin: Hebrew.
- First Use: In religious texts and angelology.
- Meaning: "Burning One" or "Fiery Seraph". In angelology, Seraphiel is often associated with the highest order of angels.

87. Seren:
- Origin: Welsh.
- First Use: Welsh name.
- Meaning: "Star". Seren is a name associated with celestial qualities.

88. Silvius:
- Origin: Latin.
- First Use: Ancient Rome.
- Meaning: "Wood" or "Forest". Silvius was a name in Roman mythology.

89. Tamsin:
- Origin: English, derived from Thomas.
- First Use: Medieval England.

- Meaning: A diminutive of Thomas, meaning "Twin". Tamsin is often used as a feminine given name.

90. Thaddeus:
- Origin: Aramaic.
- First Use: Ancient times, biblical.
- Meaning: "Courageous Heart" or "Heart". Thaddeus is a name with biblical roots.

91. Thalassa:
- Origin: Greek.
- First Use: In Greek mythology.
- Meaning: "Sea" or "Ocean". Thalassa is a primordial sea goddess in Greek mythology.

92. Theron:
- Origin: Greek.
- First Use: Ancient Greece.
- Meaning: "Hunter" or "Hunt". Theron is a name associated with strength and hunting prowess.

93. Thistle:
- Origin: English.
- First Use: Modern name.
- Meaning: Named after the flowering plant with prickly leaves and a distinctive flower head.

94. Tindra:
- Origin: Scandinavian.
- First Use: Modern name.
- Meaning: "Twinkle" or "Sparkle". It's a name associated with the shimmering quality of light.

95. Ulysses:
- Origin: Latinized form of the Greek name Odysseus.
- First Use: Ancient Greece.

- Meaning: Possibly derived from Greek "odyssomai", meaning "to hate" or "to be wroth". Ulysses is a legendary hero in Greek mythology.

96. Uriah:
- Origin: Hebrew.
- First Use: Ancient times, biblical.
- Meaning: "God is my light" or "The Lord is my light". Uriah is a name with biblical roots.

97. Uriel:
- Origin: Hebrew.
- First Use: In religious texts and angelology.
- Meaning: "God is my light" or "Fire of God". Uriel is an archangel in various religious traditions.

98. Vanya:
- Origin: Russian.
- First Use: Russian name.
- Meaning: A diminutive of Ivan, meaning "God is gracious".

99. Vespera:
- Origin: Latin.
- First Use: Modern name.
- Meaning: "Evening" or "Evening Star". It's a poetic and celestial name.

100. Wyndham:
- Origin: English.
- First Use: Medieval England.
- Meaning: "From the Windy Village". It's a locational surname that has been used as a given name.

101. Wystan:
- Origin: Old English.
- First Use: Anglo-Saxon England.
- Meaning: "Battle Stone" or "Battle Friend". It's an Old English name with warrior-like connotations.

102.   Xander:
- Origin: Greek.
- First Use: Modern name.
- Meaning: Diminutive of Alexander, meaning "Defender of the People".

103.   Xanthe:
- Origin: Greek.
- First Use: Ancient Greece.
- Meaning: "Yellow", "Blonde", or "Fair-Haired". It's a name associated with a golden or blonde appearance.

104.   Xiomara:
- Origin: Spanish.
- First Use: Modern name.
- Meaning: "Ready for Battle". It's a name with Spanish and Germanic roots.

105.   Yara:
- Origin: Arabic.
- First Use: Middle Eastern and Brazilian cultures.
- Meaning: "Small Butterfly" or "Water Lady". In Brazilian mythology, Yara is a water goddess.

106.   Ysolde:
- Origin: Old High German.
- First Use: Medieval literature.
- Meaning: A variant of Isolde. In Arthurian legend, Isolde is a tragic heroine.

107.   Zenobia:
- Origin: Greek.
- First Use: Ancient Greece.
- Meaning: Uncertain, possibly "Life of Zeus" or "Zenith of Life". Zenobia was a queen in the ancient Palmyrene Empire.

108.   Zephyr:
- Origin: Greek.
- First Use: Ancient Greece.
- Meaning: "West Wind" or "Gentle Breeze". Zephyr is a name associated with a light and pleasant wind.

109.   Zephyra:
- Origin: Greek.
- First Use: Modern name.
- Meaning: Feminine form of Zephyr, also meaning "West Wind" or "Gentle Breeze".

110.   Zephyrine:
- Origin: Greek.
- First Use: Modern name.
- Meaning: Feminine form of Zephyr, meaning "West Wind" or "Gentle Breeze".

111.   Zinnia:
- Origin: German.
- First Use: Modern name.
- Meaning: Named after the Zinnia flower. The flower is often associated with thoughts of absent friends or lasting affection.

Top 10 Shortlist of Names

1…………………………......

2…………………………......

3…………………………......

4…………………………......

5…………………………......

6…………………………......

7…………………………......

8…………………………......

9…………………………......

10…………………………......

Printed in Great Britain
by Amazon